Essential Oils

30 Essential Oil Recipes for All Occasions

Table of content

Introduction

No matter the present day human will label technology to be the greatest miracle of this century, but in reality, like all the previous timelines, nature and its various creations, stand out as the biggest and most momentous creations of this century. It is because of these creations that the modern man is able to experiment and play with various versions of utility, even the latest automated technology, takes a lead from the wisdom of nature. Technology can be short lived but nature is eternal.

A lot of people are now getting a turn towards attaining the solutions to their problems from nature. It is because the extensive use of artificial ingredients and processing technology has created a dilemma for human race, where various aftermaths can be seen in term of compromised health issues and other effects. After decade of extensive research essential oils have appeared to be the hidden miracles.

These few drops of essential oils, extracted from various plants and herbs can bring out phenomenal changes in the health and body of human beings. These essential oils can be used as a medicine, as a tonic as well as an ingredient of various recipes. There are plenty of companies which deal in the production of essential oil.

You can use essential oils at home and this book is about guiding you for this. The recipes have been listed, which can be easily followed at home without much input or budgetary investment, so that you make these useful oils more useful by making them in a lesser budget.

Chapter 1 – Few drops, greatest miracles- Essential oils

Nature has not only created the human in the best possible form, but it has also created million of utilities in the internal and external environment to make the human survive easily. These creations include various resources and natural ingredients. Everything in nature forms a corresponding and connecting role, for human utility and wellbeing and essential oils are surely a major part of our profound association to the world of nature's miracles.

One such miracle is the vast assortment of essential oils, present in different kinds of herbs and shrubs which make us believe in the wisdom of nature. They have a vast reservoir of useful substances which will cure different health issues and body problems, in the most natural way.

What is "essential" about these oils?

Essential oils are the liquids, mostly in the oily form, which are extracted from different parts of herbs and plants. These are actually organic compounds and the natural liquids, which are naturally present in different herbs and plants. As far as the chemical composition of essential oil, is concerned, these are usually made of hundreds of different compounds.

So they are truly complex in chemical nature. May be this complex nature makes them so useful for variable purposes. Whether it's a tree, flower, shrub, plant or root, there is always presence of these oils, which makes them "essential" part of different botanical species.

These are termed "essential" because survival and existence of herbs and plants rests on the presence of these oils. The different kinds of biological and chemical functions and cycles taking place in plant body will end up in absence of these oils.

But as the research about these essential oils has extended, it has been revealed that they are equally significant in solving different health and body issues of human body. Essential oils are anti-viral, anti-bacterial, anti- inflammatory, anti-fungal, and supportive for the optimum function of human immune system. So essential oils can be thought of essential substances for all of us.

Chapter 2 –Essential oil Recipes for weight loss

1. Weightbeating Citrus Blend

Ingredients:

- ➤ Ylang Ylang essential oil- 5 drops
- ➤ Spearmint essential oil -10 drops
- ➤ Peppermint essential oil - 15 drops
- ➤ Bergamot essential oil – 20 drops

Directions:

The foremost thing in this recipe is to provide the sun beam procedural alteration in the most appropriate way. When these oils will be subjected to sunlight they will eventually add up into a complete mixture for weight loss.

Take a glass bottle in blue color. Wash the bottle thoroughly, even if it is not utilized earlier, in order to put away all kinds of infectious materials. In that bottle add Peppermint oil and leave it for three days. After this initial sun therapy add remaining oils in this mixture and put for ten more days in sun. This sun theory will make up a chemical reaction in the bottle which will eventually end up to a weight loss mixture.

2. Herbal mix for weight loss

Ingredients:

- ➤ Thyme essential oil - 5 drops
- ➤ Oregano essential oil - 25 drops
- ➤ Marjoram essential oil - 4 drop
- ➤ Bergamot essential oil – 20 drops

Directions:

Take a nonstick pan and make sure that it is free of any water drops. Water drops will not allow oil to cook gently. Switch on the heater at a very low flame and put the pan at this at the flame. When the pan gets heated, add Oregano oil and cook for just few seconds. Shift it in a glass bottle. Now in this bottle add remaining oils. Use this mixture at the time when you feel hunger pangs in your stomach; use it as an inhaler as it will act to suppress the hunger pangs.

3. Weight shedding Basil essential oil

Ingredients:

- Thyme essential oil - 5 drop
- Oregano essential oil - 25 drops
- Marjoram essential oil - 4 drop
- Basil essential oil – 15 drops

Directions:

Take a glass bottle to make up a mixture of the oils. Put this bottle in sunlight for few hours. This mixture of oil can be used one drop each time, thrice a day after every meal, which will help you to burn the excessive fat quickly.

4. Bergamot essential oil used in weight loss

Ingredients:

- ➢ Thyme essential oil - 5 drops
- ➢ Marjoram essential oil – 20 drops
- ➢ Lemon essential oil - 2 drops
- ➢ **Bergamot** essential oil - 20 drops

Directions:

In a large pan add the designated quantity of water keep the flame very low. Heat water by keeping it covered when you start seeing the water bubbles coming out, remove the lid off. Cook water until water quantity is reduced to half now add sandal oil and keep heating. In the mixture add Thyme and Lemon essential oil and cook well till water is reduced to quarter part of the original quantity. Let the mixture dry and add Bergamot. Mix the two mixtures well and put in sunlight for almost three days. Shift in a glass bottle and use once daily.

5. Weight defeating Clary Sage essential oil

Ingredients:

- ➤ Marjoram essential oil - 2 drops
- ➤ Lemon essential oil – 8 drops
- ➤ Clary Sage essential oil - 25 drops

Directions:

Take a nonstick pan and make sure that it is free of any water drops. Water drops will not allow oil to cook gently. Switch on the heater at a very low flame and put the pan at this at the flame. When the pan gets heated, add Clary Sage essential oil and cook for just few seconds. Shift it in a glass bottle. Now in this bottle add remaining oils. Use this mixture two times a day after having a heavy meal. You can also use it thrice if you have a long way to go.

6. Get slimmer with Dill seed essential oil

Ingredients:

- Peppermint oil - 2 drops
- Marjoram essential oil- 6 drops
- Dill seed essential oil - 25 drops
- Bergamot essential oil – 20 drops

Directions:

The foremost thing in this recipe is to provide the sun beam procedural alteration in the most appropriate way. When these oils will be subjected to sunlight they will eventually add up into a complete mixture for weight loss.

Take a glass bottle in blue color. Wash the bottle thoroughly, even if it is not utilized earlier, in order to put away all kinds of infectious materials. In that bottle add Dill seed oil and leave it for three days. After this initial sun therapy add remaining oils in this mixture and put for ten more days in sun. This sun theory will make up a chemical reaction in the bottle which will eventually end up to a weight loss mixture. Use this weight beating blend two times a day and you will ultimately see a miraculous change in body weight.

7. Weight loss with Fennel essential oil

Ingredients:

- Thyme leaves (minced) – 1/4 cup
- Ginger (minced) - 2 inches piece
- Fennel essential oil - 20 drops

Directions:

Take a large pan and add a few drops of some base oil like olive oil in it when the oil gets heated ad thyme leaves and let them cook until they start producing cracking sound. Now in this mixture add minced ginger and mix it thoroughly. It will form a paste like substance. Take a spoon full of this mixture and put it in a glass bottle. In that glass bottle pour Fennel essential oil over the mixture and let it settle down for almost ten hours. After the recommended time use a strainer to separate the mixture and separate out oil. Put this oil in a bottle for daily use. Use it twice a day after meal, to attack the extra fat in your body.

8. Ginger essential oil for defeating extra pounds

Ingredients:

- ➤ Thyme essential oil - 3 drops
- ➤ Peppermint essential oil – 2 drops
- ➤ Ginger essential oil - 25 drops
- ➤ Cinnamon powder– 1/4 teaspoon

Directions:

Take a glass bottle to make up a mixture of the oils. Put this bottle in sunlight for few hours. This mixture of oil can be used one drop each time, thrice a day after every meal, which will help you to burn the excessive fat quickly.

9. Weight loss Grapefruit essential oil

Ingredients:

- ➢ Thyme essential oil – 5 drops
- ➢ Marjoram essential oil - 3 drop
- ➢ Grapefruit essential oil - 20 drops
- ➢ Bergamot essential oil - 10 drops

Directions:

In a large pan add the designated quantity of water keep the flame very low. Heat water by keeping it covered when you start seeing the water bubbles coming out, remove the lid off. Cook water until water quantity is reduced to half now add sandal oil and keep heating. In the mixture add Thyme essential oil and Grapefruit oil and cook well till water is reduced to quarter part of the original quantity. Let the mixture dry and add Grape fruit oil. Mix the two mixtures well and put in sunlight for almost three days.

10. Weight loss with Lemon essential oil

Ingredients:

- Water- 3 cups
- Slat–1//4 teaspoon
- Rosemary leaves (minced) – ½ cup
- Mint leaves (minced)– 3 tablespoons
- Lemon essential oil - 15 drops

Directions:

Take a large pan and add a few drops of some base oil like olive oil in it when the oil gets heated add rosemary leaves and let them cook until they start producing cracking sound. Now in this mixture add salt and mint leaves and mix it thoroughly. It will form a paste like substance. Take a spoon full of this mixture and put it in a glass bottle. In that glass bottle pour Fennel essential oil over the mixture and let it settle down for almost ten hours. After the recommended time use a strainer to separate the mixture and separate out oil. Put this oil in a bottle for daily use. Use it twice a day after meal, to attack the extra fat in your body.

Chapter 3 –Essential oil Recipes for medicinal purposes

11. Marjoram essential oil

Ingredients:

- ➢ Vanilla essence – 20 drops
- ➢ Marjoram essential oil – 15 drops
- ➢ Lemon essential oil – 25 drop
- ➢ Bergamot essential oil – 20 drops

Directions:

Take a glass bottle to make up a mixture of the oils. Put this bottle in sunlight for few hours. When you think that oils are thoroughly mixed you can put it in spray bottle and use it as an inhaler in case of asthmatic attacks and congestions. It can also be used in case of nausea and heart burning.

12. Oregano essential oil

Ingredients:

- Ylang Ylang oil – 25 drops
- Oregano essential oil - 25 drops
- Marjoram essential oil - 20 drops
- Lemon Juice -10 drops

Directions:

The foremost thing in this recipe is to provide the sun beam procedural alteration in the most appropriate way. When these oils will be subjected to sunlight they will eventually add up into a complete mixture for weight loss.

Take a glass bottle in blue color. Wash the bottle thoroughly, even if it is not utilized earlier, in order to put away all kinds of infectious materials. In that bottle add Oregano essential oil and leave it for three days. After this initial sun therapy add remaining oils in this mixture and put for ten more days in sun. This sun theory will make up a chemical reaction in the bottle which will eventually end up to a weight loss mixture. Use this blend for different types of medicinal issue like sore throat, bacterial infections and fungal infections.

13. Patchouli essential oil

Ingredients:

- Water- 3 cups
- Thyme essential oil - 20 drops
- Patchouli essential oil - 30 drops
- Mint leaves (minced) - 2 teaspoons
- Lemon essential oil – 20 drops

Directions:

Take a nonstick pan and make sure that it is free of any water drops. Water drops will not allow oil to cook gently. Switch on the heater at a very low flame and put the pan at this at the flame. When the pan gets heated, add water and boil gently, then add Patchouli oil and cook for just few seconds. Shift it in a glass bottle. Now in this bottle add remaining oils. Use this mixture at the time of headaches, vomiting and nausea.

14. Oregano Peppermint mixture

Ingredients:

- Table salt - 2 teaspoons
- Peppermint essential oil – 25 drops
- Oregano essential oil - 25 drops
- Honey – 4 teaspoons

Directions:

In a large pan add the designated quantity of water keep the flame very low. Heat water by keeping it covered when you start seeing the water bubbles coming out, remove the lid off. Cook water until water quantity is reduced to half now add sandal oil and keep heating. In the mixture add honey and salt and cook well till water is reduced to quarter part of the original quantity. Let the mixture dry and add Peppermint and Oregano oil. Mix the two mixtures well and put in sunlight for almost three days. Shift in a glass bottle

15. Peppermint essential oil

Ingredients:

- ➢ Peppermint essential oil - 15 drops
- ➢ Lemon oil – 15 drops
- ➢ Honey- 1 teaspoon
- ➢ Thyme essential oil - 1 drop

Directions:

Take a glass bottle to make up a mixture of the oils. Put this bottle in sunlight for few hours. Whenever you have to use this mixture add a teaspoon of honey in it. This mixture of oil can be used one drop each time for fat burning, digestion problems, congestion, diarrhea and other intestinal infections.

16. Rosemary essential oil

Ingredients:

- Thyme essential oil – 25 drops
- Rosemary essential oil - 25 drops
- Ginger – 5 inches
- Baking soda – ¼ teaspoons

Directions:

Take a large pan and add a few drops of some base oil like olive oil in it when the oil gets heated ad thyme leaves and let them cook until they start producing cracking sound. Now in this mixture add minced ginger and mix it thoroughly. It will form a paste like substance. Take a spoon full of this mixture and put it in a glass bottle. In that glass bottle pour Thyme and rosemary essential oil over the mixture and let it settle down for almost ten hours. After the recommended time use a strainer to separate the mixture and separate out oil. Put this oil in a bottle for daily use. You can use it in influenza, viral infections, bacterial infections and body pain.

17. Sandalwood essential oil

Ingredients:

- Water- 1 cup
- Vanilla essential oil - 2 drops
- Sandalwood essential oil - 25 drops
- Salt – ¼ teaspoons
- Honey – 5 teaspoons

Directions:

In a large pan add the designated quantity of water keep the flame very low. Heat water by keeping it covered when you start seeing the water bubbles coming out, remove the lid off. Cook water until water quantity is reduced to half now add sandal oil and keep heating. In the mixture add honey and salt and cook well till water is reduced to quarter part of the original quantity. Let the mixture dry and add vanilla oil. Mix the two mixtures well and put in sunlight for almost three days. Shift in a glass bottle

18. Spearmint essential oil

Ingredients:

- ➤ Thyme essential oil -20 drops
- ➤ Oregano essential oil - 15 drops
- ➤ Marjoram essential oil - 5 drops
- ➤ Bergamot essential oil – 25 drops
- ➤ Spearmint essential oil- 10 drops

Directions:

The foremost thing in this recipe is to provide the sun beam procedural alteration in the most appropriate way. When these oils will be subjected to sunlight they will eventually add up into a complete mixture for weight loss.

Take a glass bottle in blue color. Wash the bottle thoroughly, even if it is not utilized earlier, in order to put away all kinds of infectious materials. In that bottle add Spearmint oil and leave it for three days. After this initial sun therapy add remaining oils in this mixture and put for ten more days in sun. This sun theory will make up a chemical reaction in the bottle which will eventually end up to a weight loss mixture. You can use this mixture in stomach ache, fungal infections in limbs and for antiseptic purposes.

19. Thyme essential oil

Ingredients:

- ➤ Thyme essential oil - 15 drops
- ➤ Mint leaves – 3 to 5
- ➤ Ginger piece –3 inches
- ➤ Black pepper - 2 teaspoons

Directions:

Take a nonstick pan and make sure that it is free of any water drops. Water drops will not allow oil to cook gently. Switch on the heater at a very low flame and put the pan at this at the flame. When the pan gets heated, add water and boil gently, then add Ginger piece and cook for just few seconds. Then add mint leaves. Shift it in a glass bottle. Now in this bottle add remaining oils. This mixture will be useful in joint pains, gun swelling and other pains.

20. Vanilla Thyme mix

Ingredients:

- ➤ Vanilla essential oil - 20 drops
- ➤ Thyme essential oil - 20 drop
- ➤ Salt – a small pinch
- ➤ Honey – 2 teaspoons

Directions:

Take a large pan and add a few drops of some base oil like olive oil in it when the oil gets heated ad thyme leaves and let them cook until they start producing cracking sound. Now in this mixture add minced ginger and mix it thoroughly. It will form a paste like substance. Take a spoon full of this mixture and put it in a glass bottle. In that glass bottle pour Thyme and rosemary essential oil over the mixture and let it settle down for almost ten hours. After the recommended time use a strainer to separate the mixture and separate out oil. Put this oil in a bottle for daily use. You can use it in stomach ache, tooth ache and various bacterial infections.

Chapter 4–Essential oil Recipes for fragrance

21. Ylang Ylang oil

Ingredients:

- Ylang Ylang oil – 25 drops
- Thyme essential oil - 20 drops
- Salt – ½ teaspoon
- Grapefruit oil – 10 drops

Directions:

Take a glass bottle to make up a mixture of the oils. Put this bottle in sunlight for few hours. Now add a pinch of slay in this mixture. Mix it thoroughly. Now fill it in a spraying bottle or burn it with a lamp to add fragrance to your room. It can also be used as an aromatic inhaler and especially when the room or living area has some pungent smell.

22. Vanilla oil

Ingredients:

- Ylang Ylang essential oil – 25 drops
- Vanilla oil - 10 drops
- Thyme essential oil - 5 drops
- Mint essential oil - 20 drops

Directions:

Take a nonstick pan and make sure that it is free of any water drops. Water drops will not allow oil to cook gently. Switch on the heater at a very low flame and put the pan at this at the flame. When the pan gets heated, add water and boil gently, then add Patchouli oil and cook for just few seconds. Shift it in a glass bottle. Now in this bottle add remaining oils. Use this mixture in a spraying bottle as a freshener for your room. You can also pour it over your pillow for having a peaceful sleep.

23. Mint Blend

Ingredients:

- Ylang Ylang essential oil – 10 drops
- Spearmint essential oil – 20 drops
- Peppermint essential oil - 15 drops
- Lemon essential oil -20 drops

Directions:

The foremost thing in this recipe is to provide the sun beam procedural alteration in the most appropriate way. When these oils will be subjected to sunlight they will eventually add up into a complete mixture for weight loss.

Take a glass bottle in blue color. Wash the bottle thoroughly, even if it is not utilized earlier, in order to put away all kinds of infectious materials. In that bottle add Ylang Ylang oil and leave it for three days. After this initial sun therapy add remaining oils in this mixture and put for ten more days in sun. This sun theory will make up a chemical reaction in the bottle which will eventually end up to a weight loss mixture. This exclusive blend will make up such a nice fragrance that you will get astonished.

24. Grape fruit oil with Cinnamon

Ingredients:

- Oregano essential oil -5 drops
- Grape fruit oil–25 drops
- Ginger piece – 2 inches
- Black pepper – 1 teaspoon
- Cinnamon- 1 teaspoon

Directions:

Take a glass bottle to make up a mixture of the oils. Put this bottle in sunlight for few hours. This mixture of oil can be used one drop each time, thrice a day after every meal, which will help you to burn the excessive fat quickly.

.

25. Cinnamon bark oil

Ingredients:

- Water – 1/2 cup
- Slat – 1/8 teaspoons
- Honey – 3 tablespoons
- Cinnamon bark oil- 10 drops

Directions:

Take a nonstick pan and make sure that it is free of any water drops. Water drops will not allow oil to cook gently. Switch on the heater at a very low flame and put the pan at this at the flame. When the pan gets heated, add water and boil gently, then add honey and salt and cook for just few seconds. Shift it in a glass bottle. Now in this bottle add Cinnamon Bark oils. This mixture will serve as a classy fragrance.

26. Tangerine oil

Ingredients:

- ➤ Tangerine oil- 10 drops
- ➤ Mint oil- 20 drops
- ➤ Lemon oil– 20 drops
- ➤ Ginger oil – 10 drops

Directions:

The foremost thing in this recipe is to provide the sun beam procedural alteration in the most appropriate way. When these oils will be subjected to sunlight they will eventually add up into a complete mixture for weight loss.

Take a glass bottle in blue color. Wash the bottle thoroughly, even if it is not utilized earlier, in order to put away all kinds of infectious materials. In that bottle add Tangerine oil and leave it for three days. After this initial sun therapy add remaining oils in this mixture and put for ten more days in sun. This sun theory will make up a chemical reaction in the bottle which will eventually end up to a weight loss mixture. Use this splendid blend for making your surrounding extremely fragrant with sweet smell of these oils.

27. Cloves oil for weight loss

Ingredients:

- Water – 1/4 cup
- Slat – ½ teaspoon
- Honey – 3 tablespoons
- Cloves oil- 10 drops

Directions:

Take a large pan and add a few drops of some base oil like olive oil in it when the oil gets heated add honey ad slat and let them cook until they start producing cracking sound. Now in this mixture add water and mix it thoroughly. It will form a paste like substance. Take a spoon full of this mixture and put it in a glass bottle. In that glass bottle pour clove essential oil over the mixture and let it settle down for almost ten hours. After the recommended time use a strainer to separate the mixture and separate out oil. Put this oil in a bottle for daily use. You can use as an aromatic spray

28. Cinnamon bark oil

Ingredients:

- Thyme oil – 1/4 cup
- Lemon Oil – 20 drops
- Ginger oil – 3 tablespoons
- Cinnamon bark oil- 10 drops

Directions:

Take a few drops of Thyme oil and mix it with salt. It will form a paste like substance. Make small balls out of this mixture. Now in a bowl add the two remaining oils and dip all the salt balls in this mixture. Put a burning flame under the flame and use it as a romantic fragrant for your room.

29. Spearmint oil

Ingredients:

- ➢ Spearmint oil – 3 tablespoons
- ➢ Slat – ¼ teaspoon
- ➢ Mint oil- 20 drops
- ➢ Cinnamon bark oil- 10 drops

Directions:

Take a few drops of mint oil and mix it with salt. It will form a paste like substance. Make small balls out of this mixture. Now in a bowl add the two remaining oils and dip all the salt balls in this mixture. Put a burning flame under the flame and use it as a romantic fragrant at night.

30. Ginger root oil

Ingredients:

- Water - 2 cups
- Slat – ¼ tablespoon
- Honey – 1 tablespoon
- Ginger root oil- 10 drops
- Mint leaves

Directions:

Take a large pan and add a few drops of some base oil like olive oil in it when the oil gets heated add mint leaves and let them cook until they start producing cracking sound. Now in this mixture add minced ginger and mix it thoroughly. It will form a paste like substance. Take a spoon full of this mixture and put it in a glass bottle. In that glass bottle Ginger root oil over the mixture and let it settle down for almost ten hours. After the recommended time use a strainer to separate the mixture and separate out oil. Put this oil in a bottle for daily use. When poured in a spray bottle it will act as a sweet fragrant.

Conclusion

Nature has created and bestowed every creation for the wellbeing of human race. The high level of wisdom and intellect of nature can easily be seen in different kinds of resources made for our use. It entails that there is nothing on this planet which is useless; it can be utilized in one way or the other. Nature has created these utilities, but wants human race to use these resources and explore more and more utility around his surroundings. It is the result of this exploration that all of the natural resources have been used by humans since the very inception of human civilization. When we talk about natural resources we think of water and other gigantic resources but in reality even the tiniest leaf on this planet has some utilization.

The botanical world around us is full of utilization. Not only these botanical species are largely being used as edibles and medicinal ingredients but the oils of different plants and herbs are also having a large reservoir of utility. Essential oils are largely getting fame in various regions of the world, because of their utility for innumerable purposes. They are nature's purest gift for human race which need to be utilized in a wise and intelligent way.

In this book only few of the recipes have been mentioned, to give an assorted view of the utility of essential oils. These recipes are the simplest one which can make you prepare best possible essential oils at home. When you will learn to prepare these basic essential oils, it will be easy to prepare other types of oils as well.

FREE Bonus Reminder

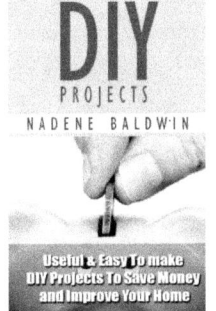

If you have not grabbed it yet, please go ahead and download your special bonus report *"DIY Projects. 13 Useful & Easy To Make DIY Projects To Save Money & Improve Your Home!"*
Simply Click the Button Below

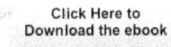

OR **Go to This Page**
http://diyhomecraft.com/free

BONUS #2: More Free Books
Do you want to receive more Free Books?
We have a mailing list where we send out our new Books when they go free on Kindle. Click on the link below to sign up for Free Book Promotions.
=> Sign Up for Free Book Promotions <=

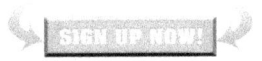

OR Go to this URL
http://zbit.ly/1WBb1Ek

www.ingramcontent.com/pod-product-compliance
Lightning Source LLC
Chambersburg PA
CBHW061934280526
45787CB00004B/1598

* 9 7 8 1 5 4 8 0 5 8 7 9 1 *